Heal Yourself!

3 Easy Steps to Discovering and Using Your Quantum Healing Energy

Concise Edition

Dr. Alexander Khomoutov, Ph.D.

LightFromArt.com

Dr. Alexander Khomoutov, Ph.D.

Cover design and illustrations by Dr. Alexander Khomoutov.

ISBN-13: 978-1983631702

ISBN-10: 1983631701

We are in an auspicious time on the planet. It is a time where the essential nature of human consciousness is evolving in profound ways. We are entering into a new reality – one that includes an awareness of our personal spiritual power, and the energetic nature of life. With this change – many people are learning to work with their energy fields to promote healing and wellbeing in unconventional ways. In this book Alexander takes you on a journey, a personal one, where he shares with you what he learned – in his own experience of healing.

In these pages, Alexander shares with you how he discovered not only his "spiritual DNA" but also the power to heal through conscious communication with it! Using kinesiology and other healing practices – he was able to talk to his body and his DNA – and learn innately what was helpful to support him in healing. Although it may sound too mystical to be true – this can be done – and Alexander is one of the pioneers who is using this information in a powerful way for healing and transformation.

Let Alexander's experience inspire you! Every human being has this power - and so do You! The time is now upon us to learn to use it! Enjoy this story of love and healing. May it open a window that allows you to expand what you think is possible – when you dare to dream!

Dr. John G. Ryan, MD
Specialist Medical Doctor, consciousness and energy based healer, University Professor, Author of The Missing Pill, and Harp of the One Heart – Poetic words of Ascension.

In this book the author shares his personal struggle to heal his own body from unexplained pain.
On his journey he learns a number of techniques that enable him to connect with his Spiritual DNA guidance.

"How to Heal Yourself" will give the readers tremendous insights into how our subconscious mind can be a guiding force leading us down the path of making good positive decisions about our health, happiness, and wellbeing.

Dianne Nassr
An energy healer and contributing author of the book A Juicy, Joyful Life: Inspiration from Women Who Have Found the Sweetness in Every Day.

Dedication

This book is dedicated to my wife Elena and angel Gosha. They inspired me to write this book.

The book is dedicated to all of you who are open to discovering the power within yourselves to live a happy, joyful and healthy life ever after...

Table of Contents

Get Alexander Khomoutov's 7 gifts FOR FREE

Alexander creates his art, photographs and books with the intention of bringing you quantum healing energy and good luck.

Get Alexander's 7 healing gifts:

- Healing book
- Easy step by step healing examples
- Your food quantum test tables
- Good luck energy wallpaper for your iPhone / Android devices
- Healing video
- 2 healing audio files

All free when you join his Reader's Group.
Find details at the end of this book...

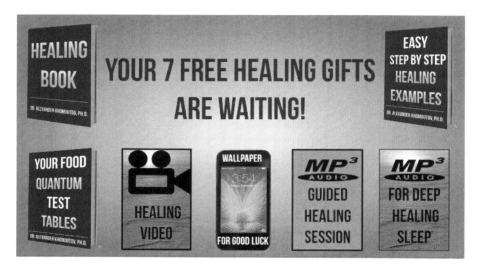

Acknowledgments

Thank you to my wife Elena. She inspired me to write this book and she was the first reader, who gave me so many suggestions.

I'm so thankful to my parents, who gave me the freedom to do what I love. They always trusted that I would use this freedom in a very positive and loving way. Very special thanks to my mother who showed me how to use the greatest power within. In 1960s and-70s she was already successfully using applied kinesiology – using a pendulum —to determine blood pressure and other things.

I'm very grateful to Lee Carroll and Kryon. Their teachings about the Innate inspired me. They gave me a magic key to unlock the sacred door to my healing and joy.

I'd like to express my very special thanks to Dr. John G. Ryan MD whose book "The Missing Pill" gave me deeper understanding of Spiritual/Quantum DNA.

I'm so grateful to Dianne Nassr. Dianne taught me how to use a Sway test when I was hosting "Healing with Lightworkers" telesummit. This is the main method I use now. She also gave me numerous suggestions to improve the book.

I'm so thankful to Janet Hofstetter for a great copy editing.

I'm very grateful to you my dear Spiritual/Quantum DNA for healing, love, joy and happiness. You were so patient to wait so long before I connected to you for the first time ☺.

I'm sending to all of you my Love, Light and Hugs.

Alexander Khomoutov

Disclaimer

The author of this book does not dispense medical advice or prescribe the use of any technique as a form of diagnosis or treatment for physical, emotional or medical problems without advice of a physician, either directly or indirectly. The intent of the author is only to offer information of a general nature to help you in your quest for emotional and spiritual well-being.

Please also be informed that any artworks, images, information from this book, etc. are not intended to diagnose, treat, cure or prevent any condition, including: physical, financial or any other problems. The information received through any of these means should not in any way be used as a substitute for advice from a Medical Advisor or other licensed Professionals.

In the event you use any of the information in this book for yourself, the author and the publisher assume no responsibility for your actions.

Introduction

Do you want to discover how to heal yourself? You're in the right place, because these easy effective 3 steps take only few minutes to learn now and can be used instantly!

Did you have any pain? I had a big moving pain in my chest almost every night for 8 months. It was so strong that I couldn't sleep. I was getting weaker and weaker every day and felt that I was going to die. As you read this book, I'll talk about the sudden death of an angel in our family — our budgie, Gosha — and how that became the turning point in my life and showed me the way to heal myself.

Finally, after 8 months of struggles, I found a very easy solution that worked miraculously for me. And I am sharing my discoveries with you in this book.

It's not just a book, it is positive energy tool to help you. A good luck energy deeply embedded in every page of the book.

The book was written with intention of helping you attract good luck energy to support your healing. Just by reading this book you are already in the good luck quantum field, if you open your heart for it. The choice is always yours.

Your first step is to read this book in its entirety. Please don't just skim through it. I don't want you to miss a single word, because it has healing energy...

The Concise Edition of the *Heal Yousef* book aims to give you a shortcut to a quantum healing method...

1. How it started

Early in 2014, my wife and I were preparing for a 3-week trip to Europe. I was so nervous and busy that I didn't pay attention to the chest pain that I was experiencing at night. I just tried to sleep with it. But just ignoring it didn't help at all. The pain became stronger and stronger. It was a very unusual, moving pain. One day it could be in one place, and the next day in another. Sometimes it moved around my chest and then it might move to my belly. By June, I couldn't sleep at all when I felt it. When I felt the pain in the middle of the night, I reached for a drink of some healing herbal tea with honey and tried to do some work on the computer until the pain stopped. Sometimes it was more than 2 hours before I could fall asleep again. But I kept up my busy schedule. I thought that a 3 km run in the morning, some healing herbal tea and good healthy food would be enough to remedy the pains I was experiencing. But those things didn't work.

I was regularly sending Good Luck energy, Love and healing hugs to my Facebook community, but I didn't take time to heal myself.

Suddenly, our family's angel, a budgie named Gosha, developed a problem with his eye. He couldn't even open it. I sent him a healing energy and asked my Facebook friends to help him. Many of them sent prayers and healing energy to him, and Gosha's eye healed quite quickly.

But I didn't ask my Facebook friends to help me. And I didn't take the time to heal myself either.

Gosha's eye was healed, but my pains became stronger and stronger. I slept less and less at night, and I became weaker and weaker.

July arrived. Time for our trip to Europe. I experienced pain during the sleepless night before we left for our trip and the next day while doing some final preparations. It

continued on the long, sleepless flight to Europe and was still with me throughout that very busy first day.
I went more than 48 hours without sleep. It was a very tough time. The next 3 weeks were exciting, full of interesting events and meetings, but still I was not getting enough sleep. The pains moving in my body woke me up in the night again and again.
Every week I was sending LIGHT & Love and healing energy and Good Luck to thousands of my Facebook friends, but I didn't take time to send Love to myself.
I did not have my usual energy, and this had a detrimental effect on our art sales. That made me anxious and fearful, which made my condition even worse. After 3 weeks of vacation, I returned home exhausted, and my pains became even stronger.

2. First attempts to heal myself

When I came back from the trip my health was very poor. My night pain had become chronic and I was 6 kg below my normal weight. I realized I needed to spend time looking after myself. I started a new routine of positive affirmations, exercise, and healthy eating.

I would repeat these positive affirmations out aloud first thing in the morning:

I'm safe

I'm happy

I'm healthy

I'm at ease

And so it is.

I started a routine of running two to three kilometers before breakfast every morning.

I made a special herbal tea with mint, chamomile, Saint-John's-wort, valerian root, ground fennel seeds, Echinacea and honey. I drank some whenever I had some pain and about 1.5 liters during the day between meals. I made sure I ate only healthy foods.

I also started to use a special device that I built myself for energy balancing. It sends electric pulses to acupuncture points.

These healing steps had helped me in the past. But this

time, after a week, there was no improvement.

I was scared. I called my family doctor. The secretary asked me about my symptoms and set up an appointment. The next day I got a phone call from the doctor's office recommending that I go directly to the hospital.

I didn't want to go there. I remembered how I had spent a half a day at the hospital waiting in line with bleeding wounds after a bicycle accident. I decided, instead, to seek the help of a professional energy healer.

3. Help from an energy healer

In the middle of August, I decided to find a good energy healer. I love the wonderful book, “Energy Medicine”, by Donna Eden [1]. I decided to find a local practitioner who uses Donna’s energy healing techniques. On the Internet I found a local practitioner. She had learned from Donna, and was certified by her to perform energy healing. A few days later I had a very helpful 90-minute energy session that helped me a lot. After that session, I had a good night’s sleep for the first time in months. I was so happy. But this success was temporary. In a few weeks, the pains came back.

I understood that only by using my inner power could I cure myself. And I have to cure the root of the problem so it won't come back.

4. Experimentation with different healing approaches

From September 2014 to February 2015 I tried many things to heal myself. Sometimes things went well for few days, even a week, but then the night pains would return. Until I found a miraculous cure. Keep reading. You'll find out soon.

4.1 Innate, Quantum DNA method

Usually scientists talk about DNA from a biochemical point of view without considering the biophysical characteristics. According to esoteric teachings, DNA has also vibrational, quantum nature. Some people call it Quantum DNA, Spiritual DNA, Soul DNA or Innate. Find more about Spiritual DNA at Dr. John Ryan's book "The Missing Pill" [6].

From Lee Carol's channelings of Kryon [2, 3] I found that we can reprogram our DNA for a long, healthy life by communicating with the Quantum DNA.

So I meditated, connected to my Quantum DNA and asked to reprogram it to be healthy and balanced to provide a long life with active evolution. In spite of this, the pain came back on some nights. Maybe I wasn't connected properly, when I was doing the reprogramming? I thought. Later in the book you will find out how to check the connection with your Quantum DNA.

On the 7th of January 2015 I realized that it could be something I had inherited from my father who had similar problems. So I meditated, connected to Quantum DNA and asked to reprogram my DNA to make me free from inherited problems.

On the 9th of January during my 5 km run, I caught myself thinking about the past and the future but not enjoying the beautiful sunny day right here in the present moment.

I switched my awareness. I felt the fresh air energizing me. I felt joy. Joy shone from inside and out of me, and when I returned I was in the NOW. I got an internal strong message that I didn't need to go anywhere to be joyful. My joy is always inside me and ready to come out, just waiting to be invited to my NOW.

On 11th of January I had the following conversation with my Quantum DNA. I know that it's hard to believe, but try to be open. I used an applied kinesiology method to communicate to my Quantum DNA. Read on to find out how.

4.2 Applied Kinesiology (AK) or muscle testing techniques

George J. Goodheart, a chiropractor, pioneered an applied kinesiology technique in 1964 and began teaching it to other chiropractors [4]. While this practice is primarily used by chiropractors, it is also used by other practitioners now, for example in treating allergies [5]. People are sometimes skeptical about whether it will work until they've tried it themselves and see the results. Applied kinesiology, sometimes called a muscle testing technique, is a way to get information from the subconscious.

There are several techniques available. Some methods that you can use to test yourself include:

- Hole-In-One Method
- Linked Rings Method
- Shifting Energy Ball Method
- Dowsing Method using L-shaped rods
- Pendulum method
- Sway Test

I tried several of these methods over a period of 6 months to find one with most consistent results. I found one method that works very well for me – the sway test. I learned it from Dianne Nassr when I was hosting the "Healing with Lightworkers" telesummit [11]. The tele-summit was packed with amazing healing information, but this method changed my life. Since that time, I have used mostly this method because I find it gives me the most reliable results. I will show you how to use the sway test. Read on to find out how.

4.3 Using the sway test

The sway test is one of the best and simplest methods to get answers from your subconscious mind, Quantum DNA and Higher Self. It doesn't require the assistance of any-one else. You must be standing to use it (see fig.1), and it takes a bit more time than the other self-testing methods.

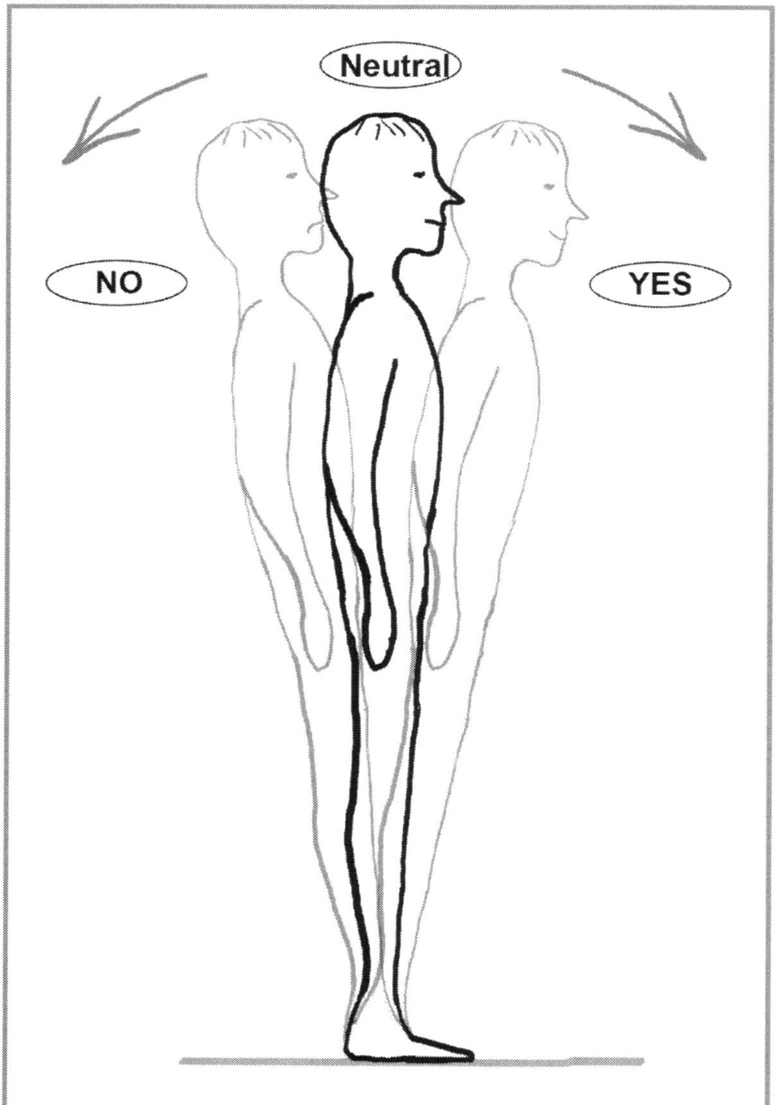

Fig. 1. Sway test.

Preparation

Use the following steps to prepare for the sway test:

1. Go to a quiet room free of distractions, including music and television.

   For me, it works the best when I am alone in the room, but you could do it with somebody else who is willing to do it with you.
2. Stand still, with your feet shoulder width apart for a good balance and your hands at your sides.

   Some descriptions of this method recommend that you face north, but in my experience I find that it works equally well facing in any direction.
3. Let go of all worries and relax your body. If you are comfortable doing so, close your eyes. If you find it difficult to balance with your eyes closed, doing it with open eyes is OK too.
4. Notice that your body continually shifts its position very slightly in different directions as your muscles work to keep your balance. The movements are subtle, barely noticeable, because they aren't under your conscious control.

Perform the sway test

Perform the sway test using these steps:

1. Make a conscious attempt to communicate with your Quantum DNA. Say aloud, "I'm connected to my Quantum DNA."
2. To test that you have a connection, state aloud something that you know that is 100% true, for example, "My name is <your name>". In my case, I say "My name is Alexander".

   You are giving your subconscious mind, Quantum DNA a chance to speak to you in this way. Your subconscious mind, Quantum DNA knows what is true. When you make a true statement, your body leans forward, because your body is drawn towards positivity and truth. Your body should begin to lean noticeably forward, usually within a few seconds. It means YES.

3. Continue testing the connection with your Quantum DNA. Make an untrue statement, for an example “my name is <somebody’s name>". In my case I say “My name is Elena”. As long as you choose a name that isn’t yours, your subconscious mind will know that this statement is untrue. Your body will lean backwards within a few seconds. It means NO.
4. Say “Neutral” to have your body come back to the neutral position. I do this between any questions. This is my own addition to the standard method. I find that it makes results more reliable.
5. Repeat the true or false tests described in the previous steps several times in random order to make sure that you are getting reliable results before asking the main question for which you seek an answer.
6. State “I’m connected to my Quantum DNA”. Your body should begin to lean noticeably forward, usually within a few seconds. It means that you are ready to communicate with your Quantum DNA.
7. Now you are ready to ask your main question. Ask your question in a way that can be answered with just “Yes" or "No.” Then if your body leans forward the answer is “Yes,” but if it leans backwards then the answer is “No.”

Discover about 2 great enhancements to the Sway method, 3 additional powerful methods to communicate with your Quantum DNA as well as other useful tips in my new book [12].

5. The message from Gosha: Love yourself first or die

The more often I practiced connecting to my Quantum DNA, the faster I was able to connect. I always tested the connections as described earlier.

During one session I got an unexpected message: our family angel, our budgie, Gosha, was dying. I didn't believe it, but one week later, on February 20th at 2 p.m., he suddenly died peacefully. We were in shock.

Elena saw Gosha's aura sitting on his favorite branch at night. I heard his voice several times, as if he was still at home. We wished him to be reincarnated and come back to us.

In one of my meditations I asked the question:

"Why Did Gosha die?"

Suddenly I realized that he died to give me a strong message that I have to love myself first and care about myself more, otherwise I'll die.

Now I realized that I was in pain for more than 8 months, because I didn't do this. Any powerful healing method will fail if I do not love myself first. So I have to change my bad habits now and then I can bring more love to others.

I took Gosha's strong message to heart. I started to develop a new habit of loving myself first, then sharing my love with others. It sounds easy, but in reality it is a very difficult task, at least it was for me. When you are doing some exciting projects or you are very busy, it is easy to ignore your own needs. Sound familiar? I remembered the preparation for our overseas trip and the sleepless night just before we left. I remembered preparing for important exams.

So I decided to work hard to develop new habits. I also needed to improve my health as the base for the rest of the changes that I needed to make in my life. I felt that I needed some direction.

So I decided to consult with my Quantum DNA about the food I ate.

I initiated connection and tested it as described in chapter 4.3 and started the following conversation.

> *Me: Is a millet porridge good for me to eat now?*
> *Quantum DNA: Yes.*

I also asked about the following foods and got the answer YES from my Quantum DNA: nori, kelp, vermicelli brown rice, brown rice, white rice, popped rice, quinoa, Alaskan Pollack, bus fish, soul fish, broccoli, celery, carrots, carrot juice, olives, cucumbers, pears, peaches, blackberries, sunflower seed, almonds, walnuts, filbert, coconuts, sweet grapes, watermelon, cantaloupe, sweet apples, bananas, oranges, avocados, cauliflower, raisins, prunes, beets, red pepper, strawberries, grape oil, olive oil, rye bread, cabbage, kefir from 3.5% milk, cheese, feta, bakers cheese.

> *Me: Is a buckwheat porridge good for me to eat now?*
> *Quantum DNA: No.*

I also asked about the following foods and got the answer NO from my Quantum DNA: butter, meat, borodinskii bread, sour cream, oatmeal, smoked sprats, smoked sturgeon fish, maple walnut ice-cream, potatoes chips, chocolate, coffee, black tea, eggs, salmon, tilapia, cod, chicken, goose, turkey, raspberries, lemons, milk, cream, cottage cheese, tomato juice, black pepper, vinegar, ketchup, garlic, brandy.

I included this list of foods at my How to Heal Yourself book [12]. You can use that list to ask your Quantum DNA about the foods that are best for you and your family.

I also asked about the following.

Me: Are morning and evening runs helpful for me to heal faster?
Quantum DNA: Yes.
Me: Are Donna Eden's 5 minute energy exercises helpful for me to heal faster?
Quantum DNA: Yes.
Me: Is honey massage helpful for me to heal faster?
Quantum DNA: Yes.

To build a healthy foundation I decided to do the following things every day:

In the morning:

- Positive affirmations (see chapter 2)
- 2-3 km run
- Donna Eden's 5 minute energy exercises [1]
- Drink a healing tea made with 7 herbs

During the day:

- After 45 minutes of work on the computer, take a break of at least 15 minutes. Do something active.

In the evening:

- 2-3 km run
- Honey massage (10 days complete set)
- Go sleep on time. It doesn't matter what time as long as it is the same time every night.
- Always get enough sleep.

To make my working day more pleasant and productive I decluttered my home office. I also put a special metaphysical energy art painting "Opening to Love" [8] on the wall just in front of my desk. Elena created it to bring a good luck and love energy to the room. Near the front door I had a "Prosperity" art print [9] that Elena created to bring good luck and prosperity. Before the art print was just pinned to the wall, but now I stretched the canvas of the print on a frame and it looks fantastic. Beside me I placed a canvas print from my photograph "Roses for Love" [10], which I created to bring love and good luck. I framed it, too, just for this occasion. So I have surrounded myself with Love, Good Luck and beautiful inspiring art.

I also cleaned up my 2 white boards. I started to use one of them just for items on how to improve my health and for reminders how to love myself first. My office looks so great now and I have more productive days. Now I have more time to love myself too. The results are amazing since I established my new habits.

From 24th of February until 6th of March.

I got a honey massage every day, except March 1st. So I got 7 massages. For 8 days I slept well without any pains at night and felt great the next day.

7th and 8th of March.

I was very busy with preparations for International Women's day and didn't love myself enough. I didn't have a honey massage either.

9th of March.

Very early in the morning I had some chest pains again. It was a very powerful reminder, so on the evening on 9th of March I had the 8th healing honey massage and slept well without any pains.

From 10th to 13th of March.

I had a honey massage every day. Each night I slept well without any pains and I felt stronger every day.

24th of March at 12.30 am.

After 2 weeks without any pain in my chest I got strong pain in the heart chakra. So I decided to talk to my Quantum DNA.

I initiated connection and tested it as described in chapter 4.3 and started the following conversation.

> *Me: Did I have the pain because of the shift to new energies again?*
> *Quantum DNA: Yes.*
> *Me: Dear Quantum DNA could you accept new energy now and in the future only at a comfortable pace, so I'll not feel pain?*
> *Quantum DNA: Yes.*
> *Me: Dear Quantum DNA, could you clean my body of any old energies?*
> *Quantum DNA: Yes.*

I felt more comfortable just after the conversation, with some traces of the pain, but not enough to disturb my sleep.

For the next 4 days I felt very good and free from any pain in my chakras.

27th of March.

I felt some pain in the bump on my eyelid. I have had this bump for years without any problems. Some time ago, I visited an eye doctor to check on it. He told me that it was nothing to worry about and I could easily live with it. It could be removed by surgery, but I didn't want to do that at this point.

28th of March.

My left eyelid was swollen and painful. It has swollen to 5 times the size of the bump. I decided to ask my Quantum DNA for help.

I initiated connection and tested it as described at chapter 4.3 and started the following conversation.

> *Me: Dear Quantum DNA, could you completely heal my eyelid today?*
> *Quantum DNA: No.*
> *Me: Can you completely heal my eyelid tomorrow?*
> *Quantum DNA: Yes.*
> *Me: Will an application of a propolis tincture to the eye lid be useful to heal it?*
> *Quantum DNA: Yes.*

I applied it at 8.30 am. By the afternoon, the swollen area had decreased to half its size.

The pain had decreased too, but not completely. I decided to apply the propolis tincture again at 1.25 pm.

Then I talked to my Quantum DNA again.

I initiated connection and tested it as described in chapter 4.3 and started the following conversation.

> *Me: Can you completely remove the bump from my eye lid?*
> *Quantum DNA: Yes.*
> *Me: Can you do it by tomorrow?*
> *Quantum DNA: No.*
> *Me: Can you do it in one week?*
> *Quantum DNA: No.*
> *Me: Can you do it in two weeks?*
> *Quantum DNA: No.*
> *Me: Can you do it in one month?*
> *Quantum DNA: Yes.*
> *Me: Please do.*
> *Me: Can you heal any bad things in my body even if I*

> *don't know about them yet?*
> *Quantum DNA: Yes.*
> *Me: Please do.*

29th of March.

The swollen area on my eyelid disappeared and I was free from all the pain. But the bump on my eyelid looked bigger than usual, and I felt uncomfortable. So I decided to check up with Quantum DNA again.

I initiated connection and tested it as described in chapter 4.3 and started the following conversation.

> *Me: Is the bump on my eye lid bigger than usual because I asked you to remove it and you are doing it right now?*
> *Quantum DNA: Yes.*
> *Me: Please do, but heal the bump area first for now.*
> *Quantum DNA: Yes.*
> *Me: Can you do it today?*
> *Quantum DNA: No.*
> *Me: Can you do it tomorrow?*
> *Quantum DNA: Yes.*
> *Me: Please do.*

30th of March.

The bump was healed.

3rd of April.

In the middle of the day I felt some small uncomfortable pain in the chest. So I asked my Quantum DNA for help.

I initiated connection and tested it as described in chapter 4.3 and started the following conversation.

> *Me: Is the pain related to the shifting of new energies?*
> *Quantum DNA: Yes.*
> *Me: Can you heal it today?*
> *Quantum DNA: Yes.*

Me: Please do. You have my permanent permission to do all necessary adjustments to new energies but only at a pace that is comfortable for me. Could you do it for me?
Quantum DNA: Yes.
Me: Please do.

I felt good after my conversation with my Quantum DNA.

After that I had a good night's sleep. I felt very good the next day. That day I continued to ask questions about food that was good for me:

I initiated connection and tested it as described in chapter 4.3 and started the following conversation.

Me: Is salmon good for me to eat?
Quantum DNA: No.

I asked this question before, but I was hoping that something changed and answer would be YES, but again the answer was NO.

I also asked about the following foods and my Quantum DNA answered YES: three kinds of fish: bass, sole, Alaskan Pollock, and cottage cheese.

I had some strain in my left eye when reading books that day. So I made the following request to my Quantum DNA. I initiated connection and tested it as described in chapter 4.3 and started the following conversation.

Me: Could you heal my eyes?
Quantum DNA: Yes.
Me: Could you heal my eyes today?
Quantum DNA: No.
Me: Could you heal my eyes tomorrow?
Quantum DNA: Yes.
Me: Please do.

4th of April.

I noticed that I didn't have strain in my eyes after asking my Quantum DNA to heal it yesterday.

5th of April.

Our Christmas cactus is flowering today! I photographed it and put it on my Facebook page and sent my love to my friends.

I noticed that I sent my love to thousands of my friends, but I forgot to love myself again. I didn't do my morning energy exercises either.

Continue talking to my Quantum DNA.

I initiated connection and tested it as described in chapter 4.3 and started the following conversation.

> *Me: Is it good for me to drink beer?*
> *Quantum DNA: No.*
> *Me: Just a little bit?*
> *Quantum DNA: No.*
> *Me: Is it good for me to drink red wine?*
> *Quantum DNA: No.*
> *Me: Just a little bit?*
> *Quantum DNA: No.*
> *Me: Is it good for me to eat ice cream?*
> *Quantum DNA: No.*

Finally in the evening I found some time to do energy exercises (instead of first thing in the morning).

6th of April.

I had a good night's sleep. I was so happy. Thank you Quantum DNA! I noticed some small pain in the right side of my chest for few seconds and then again half an hour later.

I initiated connection and tested it as described in chapter 4.3 and started the following conversation.

Me: Could you heal my pain now?
Quantum DNA: Yes.
Me: Please do.

It was done at once! Miracle! I felt so good. I was so grateful.

Me: Thank you spirit! Could you heal anything in my body that I even don't know about yet?
Quantum DNA: Yes.
Me: Could you heal it by tomorrow morning?
Quantum DNA: Yes.
Me: Please do.

I like to eat ice cream, but my Quantum DNA answered NO. I decided to ask it again. Perhaps something had changed?

Me: Is it good for me to eat ice cream now?
Quantum DNA: No.
Me: Is it good for me to eat a maple walnut ice cream now?
Quantum DNA: No.
Me: Is it good for me to eat a goat milk organic ice cream?
Quantum DNA: Yes.

This was good news for me!

Most days I use my new habits of eating food that is good for my health. I felt better and better every day.

6. At last I feel cured

Finally, I am healthy again! On April 7th, I awoke after a good night's sleep feeling very happy! I looked in the mirror. WOW: my eyes emanate light, my cheeks are rounded, and I look very healthy. I am back to my normal weight. It doesn't matter what I eat, my weight is very stable. Thank you, Quantum DNA! Finally, I feel completely cured after almost a year!

I went to my computer to send Light and Love to my Facebook friends without first making positive affirmations and doing my energy exercises. I caught myself on it. "Oh, boy, my old habits are still trying to win, but I'm alert and watching now!" I asked my wife to join me.

Me: Elena! Let's do affirmations and energy exercises together.
Elena: I am very busy in the garden. I have to finish pruning today.
Me: Gosha sacrificed his life to send us a message that we have to love ourselves first to be able to send more light to other people. Do you want our new baby budgie, Joy, to send the same message again?
Elena: No, but I am busy...
Me: Let's at least do affirmations, then. It only takes a minute.
Elena: OK.

Hooray... We did it.

Later in the day...

Me: It's already 2.30 pm and we haven't had lunch yet. Let's do it now.
Elena: I don't want to...

Elena was busy. So I decided I'd like to love myself and have lunch at the same time.

One hour later:

Elena: I was thinking about your words. Let's have lunch and do the energy exercises now.
Me: Great! I had my lunch already. But I'll do energy exercises with pleasure.

And so we did. I felt so refreshed, as always after energy exercises.

And I went with Joy (our budgie) to write about it.

Joy was sitting on my shoulder, inspiring me.

Later, I got a phone call from a gallery. The gallery was closing up and our business relationship was coming to an end. I was very surprised about my reaction to the news. If I had received the same news a few months ago, I would have grieved and been full of anxiety. Instead, I was thankful for the 20 years of good cooperation I had with the gallery. I sincerely wished good luck to the owner. Somehow I felt that it was happening for my highest good and that a new and better source of income would come in the future. It seems my request to my Quantum DNA to help me let go of fear is working well!

I'm cured, but to stay healthy and to bring more LIGHT to the people I have to love myself first.

6.1 Three easy steps for Healing, Good Luck, Love, Joy and much more...

Three healing steps that I used are the following:

1. Love yourself first
2. Connect to your Quantum DNA
3. Ask your Quantum DNA to heal you in a comfortable pace. Be open and trust the process. Be grateful for the outcome.

I also used this technique for other things. I continue to work on the bump on my eye lid, art, joy... You'll find how I have done it at http://lightfromart.com/gifts. I continue to communicate to my Quantum DNA and Higher Self to enhance my life and stay healthy and happy.

Conclusions

I hope this book has given you an inspiration to use the power within you, your Quantum DNA and Higher Self to have a happy, joyful and prosperous life.

My healing is within me. Instead of fighting against the nature of the universe in order to heal, I programmed my Quantum DNA to heal me.

I became ill because I was so caught up in pursuing goals, achieving, and helping others. I considered myself last.

Now, unconditional self-love increases my energy. The external world mirrors what is within me. I love myself, so there is more love around me too. I give more to others than before.

Any positivity you bring to yourself, you are bringing to all the people around you. Start to love yourself, and this love will help you and everybody else, because we are all connected - we are ONE.

This book will help you start communicating with your Quantum DNA using the basic Sway method.

Discover 2 great enhancements to the Sway method, 3 additional powerful methods to communicate with your Quantum DNA, food tables and an example of how to use them as well as other useful tips in my new book [12].

Sending you LIGHT and LOVE☺.

Dr. Alexander Khomoutov

Bibliography and Metaphysical Art

1. Donna Eden, David Feinstein, Energy Medicine, 2008.

2. Lee Carol's channeling of Kryon at: https://www.kryon.com/k_freeaudio.html.

3. Lee Carol, The Recalibration of Humanity: 2013 and Beyond, 2013.

4. Ph.D. Mark G. Christensen (Author), D.C., M.B.A. Martin W. Kollasch (Editor), JOB ANALYSIS OF CHIROPRACTIC 2005, ISBN 1-884457-05-3, 208 p. Publisher: NATIONAL BOARD OF CHIROPRACTIC EXAMINERS

5. Ellen W. Cutler, Winning the War against Immune Disorders & Allergies, 1998, 582 p.

6. John G. Ryan, The Missing Pill, 2013

7. Energized for healing guided 2 minutes Meditation for good effective sleep. Video by Alexander Khomoutov at:
https://www.youtube.com/watch?v=r1b1JvGiJCM

8. Opening to Love – metaphysical art print for love and good luck by Elena Khomoutova at:
www.lightfromart.com/node/8

9. Prosperity – metaphysical art print for prosperity and good luck by artist Elena Khomoutova at:
www.lightfromart.com/node/12

10. Roses for Love – metaphysical art print for love and good luck by Alexander Khomoutov at:
www.lightfromart.com/node/97

11. Leading-edge Healing group sessions, meditations: 16 hours audio downloads at:
www.lightfromart.com/node/121

12. Dr. Alexander Khomoutov, Heal Yourself! Discover quantum healing energy, attract miracles and good luck

in 3 easy steps, 2017.
13. Dr. Alexander Khomoutov, Magic of Canada: Famous Canadian Cities and Landscapes in Art Paintings, Prints and Photographs by Canadian Artists, 2017.
14. Books by Dr. Alexander Khomoutov at: www.lightfromart.com/Dr-AK-books

An extract from the full-length book

Choose the Joy of Art for Your Baby's Room!

Bring Positive Healing Energy and Good Luck to Your Baby through Unique Wall Art

Dr. Alexander Khomoutov, Ph.D.

Choose the Joy of Art for Your Baby's Room!

Bring Positive Healing Energy and Good Luck to Your Baby through Unique Wall Art

Cover design and illustrations by Dr. Alexander Khomoutov. Images of paintings are used with the permission of the artist, Elena Khomoutova.

The New Children are arriving and they bring with them many gifts of consciousness, knowledge and wisdom - gifts that will serve to change humanity in the most remarkable of ways. They thrive in balanced environments full of love and integrity. The time to foster this is with the newborn - and this wonderful book will show you how to do just that!

Thank you Alexander for creating a wonderful resource - full of tips and tools to help you create the perfect environment as you welcome this precious new life in your heart and your home!

Dr. John G. Ryan, MD

Specialist Medical Doctor, consciousness and energy based healer, University Professor, Author of The Missing Pill

This book explains how important it is to use positive energy pieces of artwork while decorating your infant's nursery. It shows you how to test the energy, as well as, determine the type of artwork that is best for you and your child. It is well written and filled with many suggestions to help create a loving, healing, and lucky environment for your child. I highly recommend it to young parents who want to create an energy balanced nursery to nurture their infant.

Dianne C. Nassr, L.C. M.S.W.

Energy healer and contributing author of A Juicy, Joyful Life: Inspiration from Women Who Have Found the Sweetness in Every Day.

Dedication

The book is dedicated to all of you who are open to discovering the power within yourselves to live a happy, joyful and healthy life ever after...

Table of Contents

Acknowledgments

Thank you to my wife, Elena, and my angel, Joy, for the inspiration. Elena, the first reader, gave me so many suggestions.

I'm so thankful to my parents, who gave me the freedom to do what I love. They always trusted that I would use this freedom in a very positive and loving way. Very special thanks to my mother who showed me how to use the greatest power within. In 1960s and70s she was already successfully using applied kinesiology – using a pendulum —to determine blood pressure and other things.

I'm very grateful to Lee Carroll and Kryon. Their teachings about the Innate have inspired me. They gave me a magic key to unlock the sacred door to my healing and joy.

I'd like to express my very special thanks to Dr. John G. Ryan, MD, whose book "The Missing Pill" gave me deeper understanding of Quantum DNA.

I'm so grateful to Dianne Nassr. Dianne taught me how to use the Sway test when I was hosting the "Healing with Lightworkers" telesummit. This is the main method I use now. She also gave me numerous suggestions to improve the book.

I'm so thankful to Janet Hofstetter for copy editing.

I'm sending you all my Love, Light and Hugs.

Alexander Khomoutov

Disclaimer

The author of this book does not dispense medical advice or prescribe the use of any technique as a form of diagnosis or treatment for physical, emotional or medical problems without advice of a physician, either directly or indirectly. The intent of the author is only to offer information of a general nature to help you in your quest for emotional and spiritual well-being.

Please also be informed that any artworks, images, information from this book, etc. are not intended to diagnose, treat, cure or prevent any condition, including: physical, financial or any other problems. The information received through any of these means should not in any way be used as a substitute for advice from a Medical Advisor or other licensed Professionals.

In the event you use any of the information in this book for yourself, the author and the publisher assume no responsibility for your actions.

Introduction

Do you want to discover how to choose artworks that bring positive healing energy to your baby?

Would you like to know how to find art paintings and prints that bring good luck to you and your baby?

Shhhh... Do you want to discover some SECRETS that the art industry doesn't want you to know and that could save you some money?

You're in a right place, because you find all in this book now...

You could use ideas from this book not only for your baby's room but for your other rooms too...

Your first step is to read this book in its entirety. Please don't just skim through it. I don't want you to miss a single word, because when I demystify the art of choosing artwork for you, you simply cannot fail to find artwork that brings positive energy to your baby.

So, how do you choose art for your baby's room?

Do you consider the following?

- The subject of the painting or print should be suitable for a baby's room.
- The main colors should be in harmony with the colors of the furniture in the room and the wallpaper or painted walls.
- The main colors of the artwork might be different for a baby girl's or boy's room.

You are right - all of those things are important. But have you considered what kind of energy the artwork brings to your baby?

Artwork can bring your baby negative, toxic energy or positive, healing energy. See fig.1. Even if two pieces of art have similar subjects, they could have opposite energies. Read on and you will learn several methods to help you choose artwork that will bring positive energy for healing and good luck to your baby. You will also learn how to avoid art with toxic energies.

You will discover how to choose museum quality giclee paper, canvas or embellished fine art prints for your nursery. Through the use of a comparison chart you will learn an easy way to choose an art print.

I have been working with art color printing for more than 15 years, so I can provide you with important insider information that will be useful to you in choosing the right artwork for your nursery.

You will discover in this book some secrets that the art industry doesn't want you to know. You will learn not only how to choose art that brings you and your baby positive energy, but you will learn some secrets that could save you money when you buy art. You will also discover some secrets about how to choose art prints that will bring you joy with beautiful colors for many years. Your grandchildren and their grandchildren can enjoy the beautiful colors in these art prints for many generations to come. You will also learn the important questions to ask before you buy an art print and how to save yourself from choosing art with colors that could fade away in just a few months.

So read on to discover more art secrets and tips and find out why I started to print art myself instead of hiring some printing company.

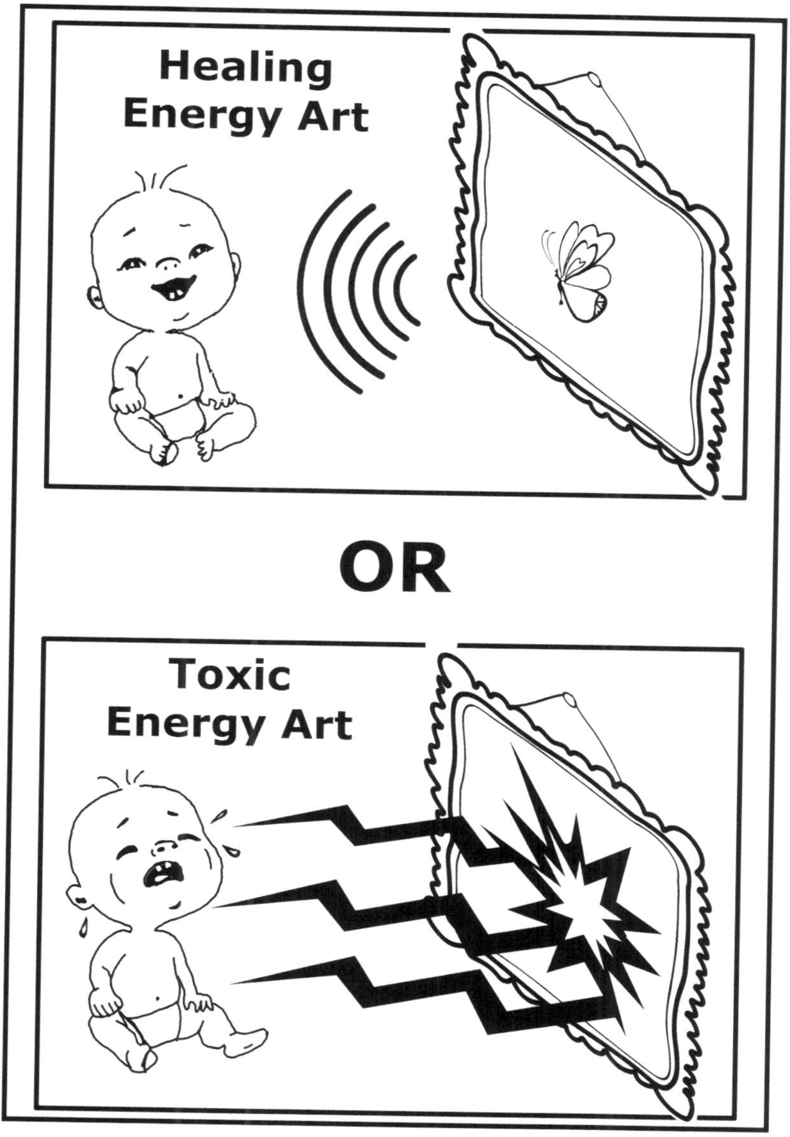

Fig.1. Artwork can bring your baby positive healing energy or negative toxic energy.

1. How to choose fine art that brings positive healing energy and good luck to your baby

When you visit an art gallery or an art exhibit, do you find that some paintings bring you joy and you could look at them for a long time? Do you find that other paintings give you uncomfortable sensations, even though they might have a pleasant subject and beautiful colors? In these two scenarios, you are feeling energy related to the artist's intent.

According to art research [1] the artist's energy is transferred to the artwork during creation. We feel this energy when we look at it. In some cases, it can bring healing. For example, according to medical research some of Nicholas Roerich's paintings bring healing to the observers. S. Smirnov investigated the art painting "The Last Day of Pompeii" by Karl Bryullov [1, 2]. The subject of the painting is tragic but the painting emanates positive energy. So the energy of the artist's intention is very important. In some cases, the subject of the artwork is positive, but it brings negative energy to anyone who spends time gazing at it. So it's very important to find artwork that will bring positive energy, joy and good luck to your baby.

Several methods are available to find out what kind of energy an artwork will bring to your baby:

- The artist's intention method
- The heart method
- The enhanced heart method, which combines artist's intention and heart methods
- The applied kinesiology methods

1.1 The artist's intention method

Let's say you found some artworks that you like. Try using the artist's intention method first. Before making your decision, do some internet research to find out more about the type of art you are looking for and the artist who created it. To understand the artist's intention in general, visit the artist's website and read the artist's statement.

What do you think about the following artist's statement?

> *Do you want more good luck, happiness, love, healing and rejuvenation? Then metaphysical positive energy art paintings, paper or canvas art prints, healing books by Ottawa artists and authors are for you.*

Yes, you are right, the artist's intention is to bring you positive energy and good luck through the art. Then what is the next step? Explore artworks on the artist's website and find some that you like. After that, read the story about each one that you have chosen and find out what the artist's intention was while he or she created it.

What do you think about the following artist's intention for a particular art painting?

> *Artist's intention: To create art to help you in discovering and using the amazing power within yourself to bring you joy, good luck and...*

While examining artworks, you may find some that look very promising. Find another one by the same artist and see if both of them were created to bring positive energy, then choose the one that you like more.

If you are just starting your search for the art, copy the above whole artist statement or the artist intention and paste it as your internet search. You will find the positive energy art images. Then choose the one you like most. That's it.

I was planning to show you real examples of art and artists' statements that emanate a negative energy. I found such artworks. When I opened the web pages I immediately felt uncomfortable sensations and I even developed a headache. My only wish was to close those webpages at once. So I decided that my book will focus only on positive energy art.

Sometimes, big gallery websites do not have enough information about their paintings or artists, so it's not easy to make a decision. In this case, search for the artists' own websites to find out more about them and understand their intentions.

What if you find an artist who hasn't provided that kind of statement? Try to find the artist's biographical information to learn more about the artist's intention.

If you still can't discover the artist's intention, read on to find other methods that could help you in these cases.

1.2 The heart method

If you find some artwork that you like, but you can't find any artist's statements of intentions, try using the heart method.

Use the following steps to use the heart method:

8. Go to a quiet room free of distractions like music or television.

   For me, it works best when I'm alone in the room, but you could do it with somebody else who is willing to do it with you.
9. Stand still or sit down in your favorite chair.
10. Let go of all worries and relax your body. If you are comfortable doing so, close your eyes. If you find it difficult to do with your eyes closed, doing it with your eyes open is OK too.
11. Put your right hand on your chest at your heart area.
12. Take 3 deep breaths, focusing your attention on your heart area.
13. Ask aloud "Dear heart! Does <title of the artwork you are checking, for example: "Multidimensional Eternal Bliss"> bring me and my baby positive energy and good luck? Thank you".
14. Sense what you feel. Do you have some pleasant comfortable sensations, maybe even goosebumps? Then the answer is Yes. Otherwise the answer is No.

To practice this method, say aloud statements about something that you know is 100% true, for example, "Dear heart! My name is <your name>. Thank you". In my case, I say "Dear heart! My name is Alexander. Thank you".

Then, sense what you feel. You could have some unique sensations. Remember them. Then, when you ask the question about the artwork, notice whether you have similar sensations indicating that the answer is YES.

Try asking aloud something that you know that is 100% false, for example, "Dear heart! My name is <somebody's name>. Thank you". In my case, I say "Dear heart! My name is Elena. Thank you".

Then sense what you feel. Remember the sensations. When you ask questions about artwork and you have similar sensations, the answer is No.

The more you practice this technique, the more reliable it becomes.

1.3 The enhanced heart method

If you are using the artist's intention method and you are still not sure what kind of energy the artwork will bring to you and your baby, add the artist's intention and the heart methods together. I call it the enhanced heart method.

Using this method you could have more reliable results. This is especially true when you are buying prints that are not created by the artist themselves. Sometimes they are mass-produced using cheap labor to make art prints cheaper. Do you know what kind of energy this process will add? I don't know either. So the first method could fail if you will rely solely on it. The enhanced heart method will give you more reliable answers.

If you could buy prints printed by the artists themselves, then you could use the artist's intention method, which is the best option.

For example, we print all our limited-edition prints ourselves and send them directly to our customers. In this case, we ensure quality and the energy of artwork remains intact in the prints. However, if you can't buy directly from the artist, another option is to buy prints done by local companies on behalf of the artist.

The more you practice, the more reliable your answers will be. Does this method work for everybody? For some people it will work just fine. For others it will not. For me, I've found that the most reliable method is the Applied Kinesiology method. I'm also using it in my healing practice. I wrote a book about it - "Heal Yourself" [3].

Read on and you will find more about Applied Kinesiology methods. Every person is unique, so find the method that is most reliable for you and use it. The more you use it, the more reliable your results.

1.4 Quantum methods

In sections 1.1 to 1.3 I explained how to choose fine art to bring positive healing energy and good luck to your baby's room. If you want to open your heart to learn new quantum ways of choosing art, keep reading! Quantum methods can be used not only to find out the energy of artworks, but also in your personal healing, and in many other aspects of your life. Feel free to skip the following chapter if the methods already discussed work fine for you. In that case, jump right to chapter 2.

1.4.1 Introduction to a quantum DNA method

Usually scientists talk about DNA from a biochemical point of view without considering the biophysical characteristics. According to esoteric teachings, DNA has also vibrational, quantum nature. Some people call it Quantum DNA, Spiritual DNA, Soul DNA or Innate. Find more about Quantum DNA at Dr. John Ryan's book "The Missing Pill" [4] and from Lee Carol's channelings of Kryon [5, 6].

1.4.2 Applied Kinesiology (AK) or muscle testing techniques

George J. Goodheart, a chiropractor, pioneered an applied kinesiology technique in 1964 and began teaching it to other chiropractors [7]. While this practice is primarily used by chiropractors, it is also used by other practitioners now, for example in treating allergies [8]. These methods could be used in aspects of your life, including finding energy of artwork. People are sometimes skeptical about whether it will work until they've tried it themselves and see the results. Applied kinesiology, sometimes called a muscle testing technique, is a way to get information from the subconscious.

There are several techniques available:

- Hand solo method
- Falling log method
- Hole-in-one method
- Linked rings method
- Thumping on thymus method
- Pendulum
- Sway test
- Shifting energy ball method (Elena Khomoutova's method)

I tried several of these methods over a period of 6 months and I found one method works very well for me – the sway test. I learned it from Dianne Nassr when I was hosting the "Healing with Lightworkers" telesummit [9]. The telesummit was packed with amazing healing information, but this method changed my life. Since that time, I have used only this method because I find it gives me the most reliable results.

1.4.3 Using the sway test

The sway test is one of the best and simplest methods to get answers from your subconscious mind, Spiritual DNA and Higher Self. It doesn't require the assistance of anyone else.

Choose the Joy of Art for Your Baby's Room

Bring Positive Healing Energy and Good Luck to Your Baby through Unique Wall Art

Buy it:

US: www.amazon.com/dp/B07486VBF2

UK: www.amazon.co.uk/dp/B07486VBF2

Canada:
www.amazon.ca/dp/B07486VBF2

You could use ideas from this book not only for your baby's room but for your other rooms too...

An extract from the full-length book

Heal Yourself!
(Revised and Expanded Edition)

Discover quantum healing energy, attract miracles and good luck in 3 easy steps

Dr. Alexander Khomoutov, Ph.D.

Heal Yourself!

Discover quantum healing energy, attract miracles and good luck in 3 easy steps

Cover design and illustrations by Dr. Alexander Khomoutov.

We are in an auspicious time on the planet. It is a time where the essential nature of human consciousness is evolving in profound ways. We are entering into a new reality – one that includes an awareness of our personal spiritual power, and the energetic nature of life. With this change – many people are learning to work with their energy fields to promote healing and wellbeing in unconventional ways. In this book Alexander takes you on a journey, a personal one, where he shares with you what he learned – in his own experience of healing.

In these pages, Alexander shares with you how he discovered not only his "spiritual DNA" but also the power to heal through conscious communication with it! Using kinesiology and other healing practices – he was able to talk to his body and his DNA – and learn innately what was helpful to support him in healing. Although it may sound too mystical to be true – this can be done – and Alexander is one of the pioneers who is using this information in a powerful way for healing and transformation.

Let Alexander's experience inspire you! Every human being has this power - and so do You! The time is now upon us to learn to use it! Enjoy this story of love and healing. May it open a window that allows you to expand what you think is possible – when you dare to dream!

Dr. John G. Ryan, MD

Specialist Medical Doctor, consciousness and energy based healer, University Professor, Author of The Missing Pill, and Harp of the One Heart – Poetic words of Ascension.

One of the things I liked about Dr. Khomoutov's book is that he describes in detail, exactly the steps he takes to effect healing change. If he is talking about foods or herbs he used, he tells exactly what he used, how it was prepared, and when and under what circumstances he used it. This is his own personal story of how he healed himself, and as such, he chronicles how he progressed over a period of time, often like daily log entries, so that the reader can do something similar if he/she chooses. He also shares some of the methods his wife, Elena, uses, and what has worked for her.

He is very forthright and clear about all the methods he uses, where he learned about the methods, and including some special "tweaks" he has used to enhance what works for him but always being careful to say what might or might not work in your own case. He leaves it up to you to pick the methods that might work best for you, based on the choices and options he puts forth.

I also liked his reference to his budgie, Gosha, whom he describes as "our family angel," and the message Gosha brought to Alexander and Elena. Having had beloved pet birds myself, I could very much relate to the love they felt for Gosha and how deeply Gosha's sudden passing must have affected them and how important and urgent Gosha's message became.

The methods and practices Alexander speaks of in this book may take time to implement. Isn't loving ourselves first and caring about ourselves more the main message that Gosha's passing was meant to convey worth our time, if it can bring us amazing healing, good luck, love and unlock the miraculous power within us to live a healthy, happy and joyful life? The miracle of working with Spiritual DNA, the higher power within you, can have profound effects even with other problems, like (in Elena's case) ants in the garden, or many different aspects of your life.

This is a truly spiritually-infused writing, and I am sure the teachings and methods of healing the author puts forth in this book can be of great insight and benefit to anyone who is open enough to put them into practice.

Dr. Marcy Rae Lifavi, D.C., C.Ht.
Doctor of Chiropractic, Certified Hypnotherapist, Artist and Author of Eletunji, The Shiny Elephant: A Fable: Spiritual And Psychological Journey Creates Choice for A Nurturing Voice.

In this book the author shares his personal struggle to heal his own body from unexplained pain.

On his journey he learns a number of techniques that enable him to connect with his Spiritual DNA guidance.

"How to Heal Yourself" will give the readers tremendous insights into how our subconscious mind can be a guiding force leading us down the path of making good positive decisions about our health, happiness, and wellbeing.

Dianne C. Nassr, L.C. M.S.W.

Energy healer and contributing author of A Juicy, Joyful Life: Inspiration from Women Who Have Found the Sweetness in Every Day.

Dedication

This book is dedicated to my wife Elena and angel Gosha. They inspired me to write this book.

The book is dedicated to all of you who are open to discovering the power within yourselves to live a happy, joyful and healthy life ever after...

Table of Contents

Other Books by Dr. Alexander Khomoutov Ph.D.

One More Thing...

Acknowledgments

Thank you to my wife Elena. She inspired me to write this book and she was the first reader, who gave me so many suggestions.

I'm so thankful to my parents, who gave me the freedom to do what I love. They always trusted that I would use this freedom in a very positive and loving way. Very special thanks to my mother who showed me how to use the greatest power within. In 1960s and-70s she was already successfully using applied kinesiology – using a pendulum —to determine blood pressure and other things.

I'm very grateful to Lee Carroll and Kryon. Their teachings about the Innate inspired me. They gave me a magic key to unlock the sacred door to my healing and joy.

I'd like to express my very special thanks to Dr. John G. Ryan MD whose book "The Missing Pill" gave me deeper understanding of Spiritual/Quantum DNA.

I'm so grateful to Dianne Nassr. Dianne taught me how to use Sway test when I was hosting "Healing with Lightworkers" telesummit. This is the main method I use now. She also gave me numerous suggestions to improve the book.

I'm so thankful to Janet Hofstetter for a great copy editing.

I'm very grateful to you my dear Spiritual/Quantum DNA for healing, love, joy and happiness. You were so patient to wait so long before I connected to you for the first time :).

I'm sending to all of you my Love, Light and Hugs.

Alexander Khomoutov

Disclaimer

The author of this book does not dispense medical advice or prescribe the use of any technique as a form of diagnosis or treatment for physical, emotional or medical problems without advice of a physician, either directly or indirectly. The intent of the author is only to offer information of a general nature to help you in your quest for emotional and spiritual well-being.
Please also be informed that any artworks, images, information from this book, etc. are not intended to diagnose, treat, cure or prevent any condition, including: physical, financial or any other problems. The information received through any of these means should not in any way be used as a substitute for advice from a Medical Advisor or other licensed Professionals.
In the event you use any of the information in this book for yourself, the author and the publisher assume no responsibility for your actions.

Introduction

Do you want to discover how to heal yourself? You're in the right place, because these easy effective 3 steps take only few minutes to learn now and can be used instantly!

Did you have any pain? I had a big moving pain in my chest almost every night for 8 months. It was so strong that I couldn't sleep. I was getting weaker and weaker every day and felt that I was going to die. As you read this book, I'll talk about the sudden death of an angel in our family – our budgie, Gosha – and how that became the turning point in my life and showed me the way to heal myself.

Finally, after 8 months of struggles, I found a very easy solution that worked miraculously for me. And I am sharing my discoveries with you in this book.

It's not just a book, it is positive energy tool to help you. A good luck energy deeply embedded in every page of the book.

Thank you to everyone who gave me great feedback on my first edition of How to Heal Yourself. I've used that feedback to make many improvements and additions, including:

- A new Questions and Answers chapter
- An example of how to use the tables in the Appendix to find the foods that will heal you and the ones you should avoid. I also revised the tables.
- New methods of communicating with your Quantum DNA:
    - pendulum method
    - L-shaped indicators method

- An image for the shifting energy ball method.

The book was written with intention of helping you attract good luck energy to support your healing. Just by reading this book you are already in the good luck quantum field, if you open your heart for it. The choice is always yours.

1. How it started

Early in 2014, my wife and I were preparing for a 3-week trip to Europe. I was so nervous and busy that I didn't pay attention to the chest pain that I was experiencing at night. I just tried to sleep with it. But just ignoring it didn't help at all. The pain became stronger and stronger. It was a very unusual, moving pain. One day it could be in one place, and the next day in another. Sometimes it moved around my chest and then it might move to my belly. By June, I couldn't sleep at all when I felt it. When I felt the pain in the middle of the night, I reached for a drink of some healing herbal tea with honey and tried to do some work on the computer until the pain stopped. Sometimes it was more than 2 hours before I could fall asleep again. But I kept up my busy schedule. I thought that a 3 km run in the morning, some healing herbal tea and good healthy food would be enough to remedy the pains I was experiencing. But those things didn't work.

I was regularly sending Good Luck energy, Love and healing hugs to my Facebook community, but I didn't take time to heal myself.

Suddenly, our family's angel, a budgie named Gosha, developed a problem with his eye. He couldn't even open it. I sent him a healing energy and asked my Facebook friends to help him. Many of them sent prayers and healing energy to him, and Gosha's eye healed quite quickly.

But I didn't ask my Facebook friends to help me. And I didn't take the time to heal myself either.

Gosha's eye was healed, but my pains became stronger and stronger. I slept less and less at night, and I became weaker and weaker.

July arrived. Time for our trip to Europe. I experienced pain during the sleepless night before we left for our trip and the next day while doing some final preparations. It continued on the long, sleepless flight to Europe and was still with me throughout that very busy first day.

I went more than 48 hours without sleep. It was a very tough time. The next 3 weeks were exciting, full of interesting events and meetings, but still I was not getting enough sleep. The pains moving in my body woke me up in the night again and again.

Every week I was sending LIGHT & Love and healing energy and Good Luck to thousands of my Facebook friends, but I didn't take time to send Love to myself.

I did not have my usual energy, and this had a detrimental effect on our art sales. That made me anxious and fearful, which made my condition even worse. After 3 weeks of vacation, I returned home exhausted, and my pains became even stronger...

Heal Yourself!
Discover quantum healing energy, attract miracles and good luck in 3 easy steps

Among the new additions included in this revised and expanded Second Edition are:

- a Questions and Answers chapter
- 2 new Quantum DNA communication methods
- revised food tables and an example of how to use them and more...

Buy it:

US: www.amazon.com/dp/B0749C5HCJ

UK:
www.amazon.co.uk/dp/B0749C5HCJ

Canada:
www.amazon.ca/dp/B0749C5HCJ

An extract from the full-length book

Inspirational Healing Quotes:

52 Weeks to a More Joyful Life, Better Health and Motivation

Dr. Alexander Khomoutov, Ph.D.

Inspirational Healing Quotes:

52 Weeks to a More Joyful Life, Better Health and Motivation

Cover design, illustrations, mixed media artworks and photographs by Dr. Alexander Khomoutov.

When you are on the path of a spiritual messenger you understand the basic underlying principle that governs the law of creation and specifically, "how to create your life consciously" is this: "You create your life by the simple 3-step process of THOUGHT, WORD & DEED." Alexander Khomoutov has taken this foundational truth and put it into book form with his latest book, "Inspirational Healing Quotes".

This book may seem simple in concept and form but underlying this simplicity are profound truths and ways of being that transcend day to day living and will take you to a higher level of consciousness that not only allows you to be a better person but also affects all of humanity. My suggestion is to please take the time to fully engage in each quote for a full week and immerse yourself in the message so that it becomes a habit of living your life. That is my plan and I thank Alexander for this amazing opportunity and the platform of this book to do so.

If you truly desire to change your life in powerful positive ways then you must not only read this book for the Thoughts and the Words but then also take the Actions of using the quotes every week for the next 52 weeks. It will change your life in dramatic, positive and powerful ways.

Richard D. Blackstone

Award-winning author and international speaker about life, love and the true nature of how the universe works, Author of Nuts & Bolts Spirituality, and Waking up the Sleepwalkers.

While reading this book you'll find that Alexander has chosen some very inspirational quotes that will allow you to begin your day with amazing new positive energy. These quotes will encourage you to allow the energy of the quote to affect your life. The topics include joy, happiness, abundance and optimism. Focusing on one quote per week will enable you to shift your energy for the entire week. This will help develop this feeling of deserving and worthiness of joy, happiness, and abundance in your life. I recommend this book for anyone seeking a direction on how to improve their thoughts allowing the energy to ultimately improve their lifestyle. It is a wonderful addition to Alexander's other books!

Dianne C. Nassr, L.C. M.S.W.

Energy healer and contributing author of A Juicy, Joyful Life: Inspiration from Women Who Have Found the Sweetness in Every Day.

Dedication

The book is dedicated to all of you who are open to discovering the power within yourselves to live a happy, joyful and healthy life ever after...

Table of Contents

Acknowledgments

Thank you to my wife, Elena, and my angel, Joy, for the inspiration. Elena, the first reader, gave me so many suggestions.

I'm so thankful to my parents, who gave me the freedom to do what I love. They always trusted that I would use this freedom in a very positive and loving way. Very special thanks to my mother who showed me how to use the greatest power within.

I'm so thankful to Janet Hofstetter for copy editing.

I'm sending you all my Love, Light and Hugs☺.

Alexander Khomoutov

Disclaimer

The author of this book does not dispense medical advice or prescribe the use of any technique as a form of diagnosis or treatment for physical, emotional or medical problems without advice of a physician, either directly or indirectly. The intent of the author is only to offer information of a general nature to help you in your quest for emotional and spiritual well-being.

Please also be informed that any artworks, images, information from this book, etc. are not intended to diagnose, treat, cure or prevent any condition, including: physical, financial or any other problems. The information received through any of these means should not in any way be used as a substitute for advice from a Medical Advisor or other licensed Professionals.

In the event you use any of the information in this book for yourself, the author and the publisher assume no responsibility for your actions.

While the author made every effort to correctly attribute each quote to the original author, sometimes the origin is unknown.

The author has made every effort to verify internet addresses and other contact information at the time of publication, however he does not have any control over and does not assume any responsibility for third-party websites or their content.

Introduction

Do you want to start your healing now?

Do you want to bring positive energy to your life?

Do you want to have the wisdom of the ages at your fingertips?

You're in a right place, because this book gives you the instant access to wisdom of the ages and joyful artworks that were created with the intention to bring healing and good luck to you.

This is not just a book of quotations - it's a tool for bringing you positive energy for healing, good luck, and love. Use it to unlock the miraculous power within you to live a healthy, happy and joyful life.

Your first step is to read this book in its entirety. Please don't just skim through it. I don't want you to miss a single word, because each page and each artwork bring positive healing energy to you.

One of the effective ways to use this book is the following:

- There are 52 quotes in the book. First, read the book from the beginning, then read just one quote a week in any order.
- Live this quote for the whole week! Put it into action. Allow this quote to be your inspiration. Write it down and keep it with you. Read it at least twice a day.
- Choose a different quote each week and so on for 52 weeks
- Open your heart to the positive energy of quotes and accompanying pictures. Trust the process. En-

joy the results and be grateful for the outcome.

An artwork can bring you positive, healing energy. Find more about it in my book *Choose the Joy of Art for Your Baby's Room!* [1].

I have created healing art prints using some of the quotes from this book. To get a print of your favorite picture and quote, visit www.LightFromArt.com [2]. Put the print on your wall. Act on a quote and enjoy positive energy of the artwork.

Thank you for choosing my book. I'm sending you my Love, Light and Hugs☺.

Inspirational Healing Quotes: 52 Weeks to a More Joyful Life, Better Health and Motivation

Buy it:

US: www.amazon.com/dp/B077PK5J3H
UK: http://www.amazon.co.uk/dp/B077PK5J3H
Canada: www.amazon.ca/dp/B077PK5J3H

GET YOUR 7 FREE GIFTS

I create my artworks, photographs and books with the intention of bringing you quantum healing energy and good luck.

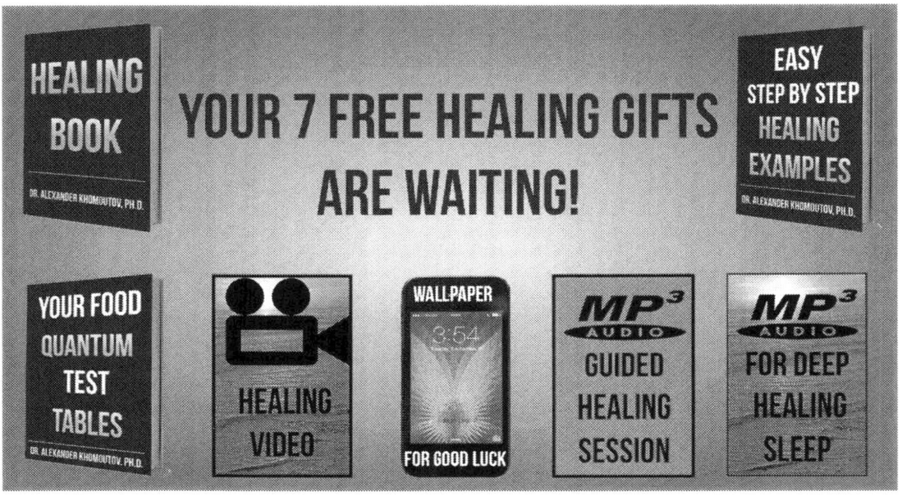

Building a relationship with you my readers is the greatest thing about writing. I occasionally send information to my Readers Group about new healing ideas and new healing books releases. You'll be the first to know next time I have some cool stuff to give away or other special offers!

Join my Reader's Group and I'll send you all this stuff FOR FREE:

1. Easy step by step healing examples: How I heal myself, my wife and more... Exclusive to my Readers Group mailing list – you can't get this anywhere else.
2. Healing book - PDF file.
3. Healing video.

4. For deep healing sleep - Audio MP3 file. Exclusive to my Readers Group.
5. New good luck energy wallpaper for your iPhone/Android or other smartphone.
6. A great healing session –audio MP3 file (about 1 hour recording).
7. Your Food Quantum Test Tables - PDF file.

Get 7 healing gifts for FREE, when you sign up for my Reader's Group.

Click here to get started:

www.LightFromArt.com/gifts

Other resources

Find out about spiritual metaphysical energy art designed to help you in your first conversations with your Quantum DNA at:

www.lightfromart.com

Discover positive energy art greeting cards designed to bring good luck to you at:

www.charitycards.ca/christmas-greeting-card-rtists/elena_khomoutova/

www.charitycards.ca/christmas-greeting-card-artists/alex_khomoutov/

www2.editionsdevillers.com/commerce/elena-khomoutova

www2.editionsdevillers.com/commerce/alexander-khomoutov

Check out positive energy Art Prints designed to bring good luck to you at:

www.fineartamerica.com/profiles/alex-khomoutov.html

www.fineartamerica.com/profiles/elena-khomoutova.html

Listen to Lee Carol's channeling of Kryon at:

https://www.kryon.com/k_freeaudio.html

Visit Dr. John Ryan's website at:

http://drjohnryan.org

Visit energy healer Dianne Nassr's website at:

http://diannenassr.com/

Check out Dianne Nassr's article in the following book: *A Juicy, Joyful Life: Inspiration from Women Who Have Found the Sweetness in Every Day*, by Linda Joy, 2010.

Watch 5 minutes of Donna Eden's energy exercises at:

https://www.youtube.com/watch?v=gffKhttrRw4

Check out spiritual metaphysical energy art prints designed for good luck, love, and healing at:

www.lightfromart.com/catalog/3

Discover spiritual metaphysical art cards for Good Luck at:

www.lightfromart.com/node/110

Discover Healing with audio group sessions, meditations: 16 hours audio downloads from Healing with Lightworkers telesummit at:

www.lightfromart.com/node/121

Healing Art

It's not just an art - it's a metaphysical energy art tool for Healing, Good Luck, Love and unlocking the miraculous power within you to live a healthy, happy and joyful life. It's created to ease up your connection to your Spiritual (Quantum) DNA for your healing and...

Discover more at:

www.lightfromart.com/node/14

Connect with Alexander

Thank you very much for taking the time to read this book. I'm excited for you to start your path to healing and to live a healthy, happy and joyful life.

If you have any questions, feel free to contact me at:

www.lightfromart.com/contact

You could follow me on Twitter: @_Alex_K

Become a fan and have a fun at:

www.facebook.com/LightFromArt

You can check out my blog for the latest updates here:

www.lightfromart.com/blog

I'm wishing you the best of health, happiness and success!

Sending you LIGHT and LOVE☺.

Alexander Khomoutov

About the Author

Dr. Alexander Khomoutov holds a Ph.D. in Building Physics. He has a great passion for writing, photography, and healing art. Alexander creates his artworks, photographs and books with the intention of bringing you healing energy and good luck. He also enjoys hiking, tennis, skiing and sending Light. His angels, wife Elena and their budgie Joy, are inspirations for Alexander's creations. Joy often sneaks into his pockets or even under his shirt and... makes him laugh ☺.

Discover more at:

www.lightfromart.com/Dr-AK-books

Get free healing videos and gifts from Alexander at:

www.LightFromArt.com/gifts

Other books by Dr. Alexander Khomoutov Ph.D.

Heal Yourself! Discover Quantum Healing Energy, Attract Miracles and Good Luck in 3 Easy Steps.

Do you want to discover how to heal yourself? You're in the right place, because these easy effective 3 steps take only few minutes to learn now and can be used instantly!

Did you have any pain? Alexander experienced a moving pain within his chest almost every night for 8 frightening months. He could sense his body getting weaker and weaker and began feeling that he was going to die. The death of a family angel, budgie Gosha, was the turning point in his life, and showed him the way to heal himself. He had an epiphany and found a very easy solution that miraculously healed him. Alexander is **sharing** his dramatic story and all of his **healing secrets** with you.

This revised and expanded edition includes: a Questions and Answers chapter, 3 new Quantum DNA communication methods, and special enhancements to Sway method, revised food tables and an example of how to use them.

Buy it:

US: www.amazon.com/dp/B0749C5HCJ

UK: www.amazon.co.uk/dp/B0749C5HCJ

Canada: www.amazon.ca/dp/B0749C5HCJ

Choose the Joy of Art for Your Baby's Room! Bring Positive Healing Energy and Good Luck to Your Baby through Unique Wall Art

Do you want to discover how to choose artworks that bring positive healing energy to your baby?

Would you like to know how to find art paintings and prints that bring good luck to you and your baby?

Shhhh... Do you want to discover some SECRETS that the art industry doesn't want you to know and that could save you some money?

You're in a right place, because you find all in this book now...

You could use ideas from this book not only for your baby's room but for your other rooms too...

Buy it:

US: www.amazon.com/dp/B07486VBF2

UK: www.amazon.co.uk/dp/B07486VBF2

Canada: www.amazon.ca/dp/B07486VBF2

Inspirational Healing Quotes: 52 Weeks to a More Joyful Life, Better Health and Motivation.

Do you want to start your healing now?

Would you like to bring positive energy to your life?

Are you ready to have the wisdom of the ages at your fingertips?

You're in a right place, because Inspirational Healing Quotes book gives you the instant access to wisdom of the ages and joyful artworks that were created with the intention to bring healing and good luck to you.

This is not just a book of quotations - it's a tool for bringing you positive energy for healing, good luck, and love. Use it to unlock the miraculous power within you to live a healthy, happy and joyful life.

Get it:

US: www.amazon.com/dp/B077PK5J3H

UK: http://www.amazon.co.uk/dp/B077PK5J3H

Canada: www.amazon.ca/dp/B077PK5J3H

O Canada! Discover Famous Canadian Cities and Landscapes in Art Paintings, Prints and Photographs

Are you ready to discover famous Canadian cities and landscapes?
Would you like to enjoy legendary Canadian Rockies, Maligne Lake and more...?
Do you want to see how Canadians celebrate winter holidays?
You are in the right place now, because this book gives you an instant joy with 73 fine artworks and photos!
Your first step is to read this book in its entirety. Don't miss a single page, because each one was created with intention to bring positive energy and joy to you.

In this book, you will find images of art paintings and photographs of well-known places in Canada, including Ottawa, Quebec City, Montreal, Mont Tremblant, Vancouver, Victoria, Canadian Rockies and more...

Buy it:

US: www.amazon.com/dp/B0739PW36C

UK: www.amazon.co.uk/dp/B0739PW36C

Canada: www.amazon.ca/dp/B0739PW36C

More books coming soon. You can sign up to be notified of new releases, giveaways and pre-release specials - plus, get 7 free gifts at:

www.LightFromArt.com/gifts

Find an updated list of new books by Alexander at:

www.lightfromart.com/Dr-AK-books

One More Thing...

Thank you for reading! If you've enjoyed this book or found it useful I would be very grateful if you'd post a short review on the book's Amazon page.

You can jump right to the page by clicking below.

US: www.amazon.com/dp/B07492FNGQ

UK: www.amazon.co.uk/dp/B07492FNGQ

Canada: www.amazon.ca/dp/B07492FNGQ

Your support really does make a difference and I read all the reviews personally so I can get your feedback and make my books even better.

Thank you very much for your support!

Alexander Khomoutov

Put your healing plan below!

Made in the USA
Middletown, DE
13 March 2020

86323838R10060